Alcoholis

The Alcohol Addiction Cleanse and Detox Guide for Dummies

Sam Peller

ISBN: 978-1-63750-047-7

Table of Contents

Introduction

Are you ready to break from alcohol easily and safely?

Cleansing and detoxification is the first stage of drug abuse recovery. It entails a period after your last drink that you devote to ridding all the alcoholic beverages or toxins within you to be able to start treatment with a clean slate. When you stop drinking, it takes up to 10 days for the alcohol to altogether leave your system. It's a tricky time. Most people struggle in the early days. You get cravings, and your thinking becomes emotional. But now there's a modern, scientific solution; changing your habits can be hard without the right tools.

The principal goal of detoxification is to securely and comfortably begin an interval of abstinence at the beginning of the healing process.

Research demonstrates the conclusion of medical alcoholic beverages detoxification, escalates the likelihood of successful treatment. Once the body is free from the short-term ramifications of alcoholic beverages, recovery will start.

This is especially true for alcohol because habits are, by definition, subconscious thought processes. Through his methodical research of the latest neuroscience and his journey, this Author has cracked the code on habit change by addressing the specific ways habits form. This unique and unprecedented method has now helped thousands redefine their relationship to drinking painlessly and without misery.

This book walks you through the detox period painlessly and explains everything you need to achieve your sobriety short or long term goal.

This book is suitable for anyone:

- If you want to quit taking alcohol for fitness and health purposes,

- If you want to reduce alcohol intake,

- If you need to give up alcohol for other reasons,

…and lot more.

Chapter 1

What is Detoxification?

Detoxification may be the initial stage of substance abuse recovery. It entails an interval after your last drink that you spend on ridding all of the alcohol consumption or poisons within you to have the ability to begin treatment having a clean slate. The main goal of detoxification is to securely and comfortably begin an interval of abstinence at the start of the healing up process. Research demonstrates the final outcome of medical alcohol consumption detoxification, increases the probability of successful treatment. After the body is clear of the short-term effects of alcohol consumption, recovery begins.

Importance of Adequate Alcohol Detox?

Alcoholic beverages could be probably one of the most dangerous substances to withdraw. As cleansing progresses, withdrawal symptoms could become life-threatening, so healthcare monitoring is vital often for misuse and dependency. As the need for actually ridding yourself of the results, alcohol is pressured in detoxification. It's important to guage for virtually any from the psychological factors that often accompany severe alcohol dependence, such as depressed feeling, anxiety, and disposition swings, since research means that such conditions complicate treatment and make successful treatment more unlikely.

Some detoxification facilities, especially luxury programs that may offer one-on-one care, may evaluate patients for co-occurring psychiatric conditions during cleansing in order that any mental medical issues could be appropriately managed.

Alcohol cleansing could be uncomfortable until withdrawal symptoms are determined. Withdrawal is most likely the most difficult section of the treatment process. Patients who've involved with heavy, long-term drinking suffer from physical reliance on alcohol consumption and depend on it to activate the body's regulatory functions.

Alcohol Withdrawal: Physical Symptoms

Patience experience alcohol consumption withdrawal

differently. However, a lot of people will experience at least some of the pursuing severe alcohol withdrawal symptoms:

- Racing pulse
- Increased blood pressure
- Fever
- Sweating
- Headache
- Mood swings
- Anxiety
- Confusion
- Agitation
- Seizures.

Seizures would be the most dangerous of acute alcohol consumption withdrawal symptoms. They happen as the human brain as well as the cellular material within it have transformed because they have become acquainted with the persistent existence of alcohol consumption and its own sedating effects on your own system.

When alcohol is abruptly removed your system, the body cannot access chemicals that assist your central nervous system calm itself after being excited. The mind challenges to improve towards the rebounding amount of activation. Sometimes your brain can't match all this fresh excitatory neuronal activity, that may result in a seizure.

The opportunity of experiencing an alcohol-related seizure peak at 24-48 hours following a last drink remains high. Occasionally, several times after that.

Therefore, it is vital to your treatment course that you focus on detox and possess all of the alcohol removed from your body first. For a few, starting treatment for alcohol consumption abuse after properly completing cleansing may be the ultimate way to grab yourself to perform sobriety. That way, probably the most literally uncomfortable part is finished, and you'll focus your time and efforts on recovery.

What to Expect

The severity from the person's withdrawal during detox is closely linked to how severe and long-standing he continues to be addicted. It is critical to be aware that your reference to detoxification can vary greatly from everything you read here or everything you might have seen in others. Precisely how your cleansing advances will be suffering from many factors, so it's difficult to determine with precision what course your detoxification might take.

However, you can get an over-all timeframe for the detox procedure, filled up with the progression of symptoms.

The Initial Hours of Alcohol Consumption Detox.

Cravings certainly are a several initial symptoms of alcohol consumption withdrawal, and a definitive indication that the body is starting the cleansing process.

- Cravings can happen within hours of choosing the final drink and continue much in to the detoxification process.

The first hours of cleansing may possibly also involve symptoms such as:

- Nausea and vomiting.

- Anxiety, restlessness, depressive disorder, or irritability.
- Spikes in heartrate and blood pressure.
- Nightmares and insomnia.
- Tremors (quite common for all people levels of alcohol consumption addiction).

For patients with a rise of extensive physical reliance on alcohol consumption, symptoms may persist and get progressively worse through the entire withdrawal process.

The First Two Times of Alcohol Consumption Detox

Following an initial hours of untreated alcohol withdrawal, more acute severe symptoms are possible. As well as the symptoms explained above, new symptoms at the moment range between hallucinations and seizures.

The symptoms that develop inside the first two times of detox could become life-threatening if your brain struggles to pay for having fewer chemical indicators to re-enter the resting reasonable health after anxiety or enjoyment and may lose its control over heartrate, blood pressure, and nervous system activity.

- Hallucinations are possible with this stage of detoxification.

- Seizures are possible aswell, mostly in the first 12 to 48 hours following last drink, but can continue for occasions following the operation starts.

- Fast heartrate and high blood pressure continue if no intervention occurs.

- Chest pain may arise, which can indicate insufficient blood flow to the guts (because of increased blood pressure and to the heart's higher energy importance).

- Delirium tremens: a severe, dangerous effect of acute alcohol consumption withdrawal (discover below for symptoms).

- For most, the cleansing process won't be closing at 48 hours.

- Severe or long-standing cases of alcohol consumption addiction may necessitate particularly close monitoring for instances, following a decision to detoxify has begun.

Additional Alcohol Detox Process

Detoxification can continue for some days following preliminary withdrawal symptoms develop, which urges, restlessness, and anxiety intensify with long exercises of untreated alcohol consumption withdrawal. If present, instead of managed carefully, seizure activity may increase in severity and rate of recurrence.

Following a first 48 hours of detox, seizure risk will begin to reduce often. However, continuing medical observation could be necessary as the opportunity of extreme misunderstandings and cardiovascular occasions such as heart attack and heart stroke remain elevated.

If individual experience these results, symptoms usually occur within 48 to 96 hours following a last drink. Sometimes, they have a postponed starting place, starting between 7 and 10 moments following last sip.

Delirium tremens (DT) symptoms include:

- Body tremors.

- Agitation or irritability.

- Fever and perspiration.

- Extreme confusion or disorientation.

- Quick mood changes.

- Hallucinations.

- Seizures.

Since Deliriun Tremen is an unhealthy condition with an increased death rate, it will always be managed in an inpatient medical hospital's intensive treatment device. Mortality rates in unmanaged situations of delirium tremens are 10-15%. Sedating medications, diligent guidance, and supportive care and attention can make a difference before health threats subside.

Risk Factors for Delirium Tremens

A guy experiencing symptoms in Delirium tremens won't develop Atlanta divorce attorneys recovering alcohol consumer, but because it is indeed dangerous, you have to have a medical doctor or additional addiction treatment professional, evaluate your risk to have the ability to best-plan potential problems. The rapidity of onset and intensity of DT symptoms depends upon just how much and just how normally a person drinks.

Risk factors for developing DT during alcohol consumption withdrawal include:

- The cessation of consuming over time of consuming heavily.
- Not attempting to consume enough food before substantial consuming.
- Head injury, infection, or illness inside a person with a brief overview of heavy consuming.
- History of alcohol consumption withdrawal experiences.
- Drinking a whole lot or often to obtain additional

when compared to a decade.

Alcohol cleansing and withdrawal could be physically and psychologically taxing health issues, cravings, and feeling swings are normal. It seems like frightening information, but it's vital that you exit appropriately; familiarized using the detoxification method, particularly if you possess a severe dependency.

Can I Take Action at Home?

Actually if you'd decide to cleanse from alcohol in the home, finding professional supervision is actually crucial. Mild to moderate withdrawal symptoms could be handled on either an inpatient or outpatient basis, as research shows little difference in results between these configurations. When there's a risk for severe symptoms, alcohol consumption withdrawal should be maintained within a severe medical establishing. Alcohol detoxification and withdrawal bring the opportunity of extreme health consequences, including hallucinations, seizures, and lack of life. Finding a highly effective cleansing program, whether it's carried out with an inpatient or outpatient basis - is paramount to your recovery security.

You will see outpatient recovery programs that let you straighten out recovery out of your home. Nevertheless, you should talk to your physician before buying outpatient detox, as it can not be the probably option if you're in risk for physical withdrawal symptoms or you have other circumstances that could jeopardize your recovery efforts.

Relatively mild symptoms of withdrawal could be managed if alert to appropriate medications and frequent check-ins using a supervising physician.

However, it really is difficult to forecast withdrawal advancements, and additional, difficult to regulate for all you factors in the home. For these and various other reasons, going right through detoxification at something and working through others of treatment out of your home is an excellent option for some in early recovery.

Alcohol Detox Treatment

Many of the symptoms of acute alcohol consumption

withdrawal could have largely faded after five times of detox, although some may persist for weeks or longer. Any severe symptoms still present at the moment will become clinically handled in the cleansing center.

Clinically assisted detoxification involves professional health monitoring through the detox phase to ensure your safety through the entire risky alcohol withdrawal effects. Traditional treatment offers you supportive therapy that will prepare you for time, for living and demonstrate how exactly to manage drinking temptations effectively.

Luxury treatment also provides quality substance abuse treatment, but these facilities additionally place focus on personal privacy and comfort. Within an extravagance or professional program. You'll find many amenities i.e. private rooms, usage of the web, leisure entertainment, and more one-on-one treatment.

Since alcohol consumption detoxification, withdrawal, and recovery can initially be this uncomfortable procedure, luxury configurations are ideal for those in recovery from alcohol consumption addiction. Many select to undergo treatment in the very best luxury home rehabilitation programs in America, where they'll also receive mental counseling and support from others in recovery.

Traditional treatment programs use similar therapeutic strategies and can end up being as helpful as luxury rehabs are towards the people in recovery. The amount of amenities could be significantly less than those at the luxury centers. However, the procedure services are usually offered at a smaller cost. Whatever your decision, make sure that you put your overall health first, both physical and mental, through the entire procedure.

Chapter 2

Natural Treatments for Alcoholism Treatment and Recovery

Alcoholism Treatment and recovery are complicated procedures that want a whole lot of constant support. Although it isn't recommended to rely exclusively on option therapies or remedies for the support, specific natural approaches might help improve your well-being while undergoing alcoholism treatment.

When is Alcoholism Treatment Necessary?

Alcoholism, the favorite term for alcohol consumption dependence, sometimes appears as several features, including craving, insufficient control, physical dependence (typically triggering symptoms like nausea and sweating upon withdrawal), and tolerance.

However, because alcoholism can lead to plenty of friendly and emotional problems aswell as serious health issues, it's necessary to seek treatment when you have any observable symptoms of alcoholism (just like a compulsion to drink or failing to limit the amount of alcohol you consume).

Natural Support

Sure natural substances and mind-body therapies show promise as a means of supporting your overall health while undergoing alcoholism treatment. If you're considering the usage of these approaches, make sure that you discuss its potential benefits and dangers using the health-care experts associated with your alcoholism treatment.

Acupuncture for Alcohol consumption Addiction

Acupuncture (an importance-based therapy long within traditional Oriental medication) is often recommended in reducing alcohol desires, relieve withdrawal symptoms, and simplify the panic and significant depression frequently experienced by alcoholics.

Certainly, a 2002 report of 34 alcoholics found that a

fortnight of acupuncture treatments (in conjunction with carbamazepine; a drug sometimes within managing alcohol withdrawal) helped decrease the participants' withdrawal symptoms. However, a systematic review published in '09 2009 figured there may be insufficient evidence to assist acupuncture's effectiveness in alcoholism treatment.

Milk Thistle for Alcoholism

Milk thistle (Silybum marianum), an all natural herb full of the antioxidant silymarin, is often touted as a means of restoring liver organ health insurance and avoiding alcohol-induced liver organ damage. While research demonstrates milk thistle may offer some advantage to the people wanting to treat alcohol-related liver organ disease, more studies had importance to attract any definitive conclusions about the herb's effectiveness in improving liver health.

Kudzu for Alcohol consumption Dependence

In a 2003 research on lab rats, scientists discovered that feeding the animals extract of kudzu (Pueraria lobata) helped curb their alcohol dependence. Also, little research released in 2005 demonstrated that taking kudzu vitamins helped reduce alcohol consumption intake in humans.

The Need for Alcoholism Treatment

Without help of alcoholism treatment, you may increase your risk of experiencing certain problems linked to excessive drinking, including:

- Alcoholic hepatitis (inflammation from the liver organ)
- Cirrhosis (scarring from the liver organ)
- Gastritis (swelling from the liner from the belly)
- Pancreatitis
- High blood pressure
- Bone loss

Furthermore, alcoholism continues to be associated with an increased incidence of several cancers, including:

- Colon cancer
- Breast cancer
- Malignancy from the jaws, neck, esophagus,

larynx, and liver.

Choices for Alcoholism Treatment

Given the significant health threats connected with alcoholism, it is advisable to seek alcoholism treatment only from professional healthcare with professional facilities.

Standard alcoholism treatment plans may begin with detoxification, as well as perhaps involve house and outpatient programs that uses many social supports.

Chapter 3

5 Methods for Detoxing from Alcohol

Alcoholism is a substantial disease which should receive medical attention. Yet, only around 10 to 20 percent of people experiencing alcohol drawback receive treatment predicated on the American Academy of Family Doctors.

Regardless of the known explanations why people don't undergo treatment, it really is vital to sobriety. So, if you are lamenting over dropped associations, money, or careers credited to alcoholism, or while you believe that perchance you drink an excessive amount of, cleansing may be considered a fantastic option for you personally. Here are some tips to obtain clean and sober and complete alcohol consumption detoxification successfully.

1) Make a concept and invest to quit

An important component in getting sober and going through detox is to create an arrangement for sobriety. While people can reap the advantages of involuntary cleansing and treatment, your recovery will primarily depend on your dedication to improve.

In such, you ought to be ready to produce a changeover from your own present life to detoxification and transition again into culture. Some cleansing programs last a few days, while some may take up to week or higher. Facilities often use medications to assist severe addiction instances, so find out about your options.

2) Understand the withdrawal symptoms.

Going through detoxification doesn't mean you won't experience withdrawal symptoms, mainly if you're a long-term or significant consumer of alcohol. The Improvements in Psychiatric Treatment journal cites that patients should be aware of what to expect through the drawback, and just how those symptoms could be treated. Knowledge may be the main element here. Common alcohol consumption drawback symptoms include:

- Depression

- Anxiety

- Irritability or restlessness

- Exhaustion or insomnia

- Seizures or delirium tremens (DTs)

- Urges for alcohol

- Sweating

- Physical weakness

3) Recognize that detox can be an initial step.

Some think that cleansing is one process, and one is okay to re-integrate into society and prevent consuming forever; this isn't quite so. Detoxification is a preliminary area of the healing process. A thorough treatment plan will make sure that detoxification is employed in tandem with additional treatment options like cognitive behavioral therapy.

4) Get new meaning in your daily life.

A deterrent towards the people seeking help for alcohol consumption is that they think their life is probably not as enjoyable without it. Experience could be fun, enjoyable, and utterly advantageous without alcohol consumption! Explore different therapies like artwork, music, pilates, or trekking to find new, healthy methods to enjoy from life. Besides, maybe it's fun when you awaken having a killer hangover, so you can't remember everything you did yesterday evening?

5) Change your daily food diet and exercise routine.

The usage of alcohol consumption and another withdrawal period can lead to a person to become dehydrated, so drink a whole lot of water. Additionally, alcohol consumption can deplete the body of essential nutrition and damage vital organs. Get your body ideal again by nourishing it with foods full of vitamins and minerals and by training. Proper maintenance of your body leaves you refreshed plus your brain clear (healthy bodywork). To create a concept to quit alcohol consumption, make a concept to nurture your body as well.

Considering alcohol consumption, detox is an excellent first step inside a lifelong intent to acquire sober. Alta Mira Recovery is certified to take care of alcohol consumption withdrawal symptoms and provide continuous care. Call us today for more information about our service and how exactly we will exactly help you to get over alcoholism or alcohol consumption abuse. Your lifestyle won't be dropped without alcoholic drinks. Your brand-new life can begin once you just forget about your dependence.

Chapter 4

9 Ways of Cleansing After a Long Night

1. Sleep in.

A hangover may be the biological taxes you get after partying. There is no actual remedy, but sleeping through the most unfortunate of it really is a fantastic spot to start out. Plus, though alcohol consumption cause you to drift off promptly, it includes you crap rest.

2. Drink a whole lot of water.

It's likely that, in the event that you went big on cocktails yesterday evening, you're probably incredibly dehydrated at this time, which can make you feel drained and cause a headache. Blame it around the alcohol because it's a diuretic.

3. Intensify the rehydration with electrolytes.

Gatorade, coconut normal water, and Pedialyte (the children's drink and hardcore partier's key tool) contain electrolytes, including sodium and potassium, that help your body to carry onto water.

4. Eat eggs for breakfast

Both alcohol consumption and mixers are high in glucose; a hangover is at large part a massive sugars crash. Your blood sugar can decrease to virtually zero. So it is important to get some good food back to the body. Eggs contain cysteine, an amino acid that counteracts a harmful byproduct of alcoholic beverages' metabolism. Can't take it in? Focus on something similar to crackers, grain, or broth.

5. Sip some ginger tea.

It can benefit quell nausea and may also reduce any lingering dizziness. Plus, it's just very soothing, drink clear water. You will need to prioritize taking enough water.

6. Add honey

Fructose has shown (anecdotally and in several research) to accelerate alcohol consumption metabolism in the body. Honey provides you an excellent fructose bang for your buck. (So eat some of that, too.)

7. Get yourself a walk and get some good oxygen.

The claims that o2 relieve hangover symptoms are sketchy at best (remember air pubs?), though many people swear the bond is real. Walk in the brand new air and get the breathing going slightly. Even more o2 moving through your veins can only support your liver organ using the monumental job of filtering out the toxins and bacteria from alcohol consumption out of the bloodstream. Plus, it'll get you out of the stuffy apartment and it will feel great to become up and about.

8. Ramp it up to jog or take part in other styles of exercise.

"Training produces endorphins (disposition enhancers), which will help you feel better faster," Beth Recanati, M.D., a women's health specialist, tells Personal. Try this twisty pilates routine for your entire day after an especially significant date to wring yourself out, as being a dishtowel.

9. Whenever your belly is made for it, eat meat, coffees, and lentils.

Chapter 5

How to Detox Alcohol from Home

When you have browsed the cautionary caution in the preceding section but nonetheless desire to follow self-detox from alcohol consumption, here are plenty of preliminary steps that are essential to attempt to guarantee the process is safe, and to increase its probability of success:

- Remove all alcohol consumption out of your home; this really is an important step.
- Crystal clear the regular, create plenty of time essential for complete detoxing, could take weeks. Make sure almost nothing stands with techniques.
- Obtain active support, finances for this with family or friends who'll make certain a detoxing person is Okay, and who'll be there if the average indivdual needs anything.
- Concentrate on hydration, make certain a detoxing person drinks enough liquid because this will rehydrate the body and be gone toxins.

- Take vitamins, B-complex, Niacin, vitamin C, magnesium, and zinc. Test to find out which work best.

Main Types of Self-Detox from Alcohol

- **Cool Turkey**: fast, abrupt, more painful means of avoiding alcohol consumption

- **Tapering Off:** continuously preventing, using less and less alcohol

Alcohol detoxification can be executed at home, however, not under some conditions.

Alcohol cleansing in the home is normally safe for the binge-drinker who only celebrate on weekends because their bodies never have developed the full-blown addiction. These drinkers could become significantly uncomfortable while trying self-detox from alcohol consumption, but likely this discomfort won't transfer towards the life-threatening category.

This is especially true from the *"Tapering Off"* approach to self-detox. Maybe it's done securely When there is certainly someone else presently monitoring the amount of alcohol consumption consumed, and If the average person is usually permitted to drink just a glass or two with a smaller alcoholic beverages content material, like ale, and If this usage is doled out from the supervisor only. If the alcohol-dependent person is left to monitor himself or herself, generally, the individual increase usage to pun intended, the pain of withdrawal.

The Cool Turkey Approach

Lady in despair addresses her face with hands seated around the couch "Cool Turkey" implies sudden secession of alcohol consumption. This system can succeed for a few because it quickens the street to recovery. It really is much harder compared to the following "Tapering Off" technique, but they have demostrated to be always a sound choice for a few.

It is critical to comprehend, however, that withdrawal symptoms could be very severe. Your body from the alcoholic knows large sums of alcohol consumption, which is why abrupt discontinuation of intake may become a surprise to the body. The Cool Turkey method could cause another withdrawal symptoms:

- Nausea
- Headaches
- Insomnia
- Sweating
- Heartrate increase
- Hallucinations (audio-visual-tactile)
- Fever
- Seizures.

The Tapering Off Approach

Tapering off is usually a means of alcohol consumption detoxification which includes a slow reduced amount of one's amount of daily alcohol consumption intake. It really is a less severe strategy when it comes to adverse effects such as stomach pains and aches, nausea, and other unpleasant symptoms. Many people choose beverage like a tapering off tool, so if one can be an ale lover, this might work within their favor. If indeed they opt as a result of this cleansing method, make sure to limit a normal alcohol intake regularly instead of fluctuate backward and forwards.

Overall, alcohol consumption house detoxification is neither the most effective nor the safest method of quitting alcohol consumption addiction; however, occasionally, it could be a cheap and effective one. Having someone around to make sure a detoxing is definitely specific and steady, and always an excellent notion, so if one chooses to endure self-detox from alcohol consumption, they need to remind their most beautiful friend, family, or simply a doctor to be certain of these regularly, in the case. That's essential if a person really wants to apply safe alcohol detoxification in the home.

Risks of Alcohol Detox from Home

The dangers of alcohol detoxification in the home far outweigh the enormous benefits for a number of reasons. Initial, detoxing in the home is seldom fruitful. Lots of people quit the task and resume consuming inside the first day, simply from the problem of controlling the symptoms. A location of concern will be that this alcoholic does not have the support in the home that he/she could possess in the cure center. There's an importance for guidance, friends, helpful mentors, and group support that's seldom within the house position, rather than present in a day per day, seven days weekly. The drinker might use essential medical attention due to the life-threatening physical and emotional symptoms that may happen during detox.

Adverse Effects of Detoxing from Home

As being a reminder why the response towards the question "How exactly to safely detox from alcohol in the home" it is vital to learn that "One can't constantly be sure it will likely be safe," Common side effects of self-detox include:

- Pacing, restlessness, and irritability.
- Agitation
- High blood pressure
- Muscle cramps, body pain, and tremors
- Increased heartrate
- Diarrhea and additional intestinal crises
- Hypoglycemia or low bloodstream sugar level
- Headaches, dizziness, and confusion
- Hot and cold flashes change of your body's

temperature.

Physical Symptoms

Frequently, it is the serious and disabling physical symptoms of detox that change the drinker's brain about continuing with the task. These symptoms have a tendency to exist severe and really should preferably be supervised by medical personnel. Some physical problems include:

- The necessity to go around, restlessness and irritability
- Feeling as if your skin can be crawling and being agitated
- Blood circulation pressure can increase to high levels
- Pains and shakes, and sense as if "every muscle hurts" as alcohol consumption are flushed from the machine
- Pulse rate raises with any risk of strain from the withdrawal
- The digestive system moves into crisis; diarrhea is common

- The blood sugars drop because alcohol is some sort of sugar in the body
- The person with average skills may own symptoms of hypoglycemia
- Headaches, dizziness, and confusion
- Tiredness, heat adjustments in the body, hot and cool flashes
- Shaking and cramping muscles.

Psychological Symptoms

There could be severe psychological symptoms as well, including:

- Generalized anxiety sense as being a hammer is dangling outrageous, and bad things have a tendency to happen
- Hallucinations
- Intense urges to get relief
- Sense like the body is usually arriving apart.
- Feel swings - from anxiety to hopelessness, to suicidal
- Paranoia often accompanies the hallucinations and

may escalate into defensive actions.

Delirium Tremens

Delirium Tremens (DT) would be the most dangerous withdrawal sign for alcoholics, with the likelihood of them occurring to at least 1 in 10 individuals in withdrawal. The death rate from serious situations of DTs is often as high as 35%.

The symptoms of delirium tremens can happen within 72 hours of alcohol withdrawal and will appear unexpectedly. DTs may appear anytime through the withdrawal period but will show through the initial ten times.

Indicators of delirium tremens during self-detox include:

- Grand mal seizures, regarded as a lack of awareness and violent muscle contractions

- Jeopardized heart functions including high blood pressure, suppressed yoga breathing, and low oxygen levels

- Hallucinations

- Paranoia

- Confusion

- Anxiety and agitation.

DTs treatment and monitoring is vital because they experience many dangerous characteristics, such as:

- Grand mal seizures, where a person might thrash about, swallow their tongue or bite it off, lose awareness, or become physically hyper-strong.

- Heart functions could be compromised as pulse rate, and blood pressure rises, and yoga breathing could be suppressed, which causes the oxygen source towards the cardiovascular to decrease. The likelihood of heart stroke or heart attack is usually increased.

- Experiencing alcoholic DTs may lead to having hallucinations such as bugs crawling on your skin or spiders in the region. They could claw at their encounters and rip at their epidermis. The average indivdual may also do long-term injury to their eye, convinced that their eye is becoming broken due to the hallucinations.

- The alcoholic could become paranoid and attack someone because they consider they might be being hunted or threatened.
- The alcoholic will be confused with the sugar withdrawal, that may result in impaired judgment in critical situations.
- The person with average skills could be anxious and agitated, struggling to cope with social situations.

Factors for continuing to drink

The main reason that folks with alcohol abuse problems continue steadily to drink is that they believe they "own it in order." That is an unhealthy thought because they will probably die from alcohol poisoning, like Amy Winehouse.

Listed below are probably the most cited explanations why someone continues using their addictive behavior:

- **Denial:** They deny the problem, ignore their

behavior, and withdraw from criticism and the ones that confront them with their addiction issues.

- **<u>Lack of control at cure center:</u>** They would like to control the problem themselves because they have already dropped control of their bodies and relationships.

- **<u>Fear of change within their lives:</u>** They fear the discomfort and pain of withdrawal and the procedure of rehabilitation. Any kind of change moves them out of their "safe place."

- **<u>Fear of life:</u>** The average person knows that they don't have the coping skills to truly have a normal life, so they select a dysfunctional pattern. It might be bad, nonetheless it is preferable to appearing inadequate.

- **<u>Self-defeating attitude:</u>** Many people who have alcohol dependency believes there isn't help and hope. These folks need important mental health treatment and counselling for depression, simultaneous with addiction rehab

- **Stigma:** Many people fear "how many other people will believe" if indeed they head to rehab for support. They don't recognize that these "other folks" they're concerned about already spot the addiction problem.

- **The wish to die:** The addicted individual has lost the desire to live and it is using alcohol to commit a kind of "slow suicide." This sort of person will drink until they die unless they receive an unwanted intervention.

- **Cost:** Many alcoholics will say that the price is usually too prohibitive to allow them to seek specialized help through a rehab center, but that is erroneous. Insurance covers thirty days of rehab, Medicare covers thirty days, and if someone does not have any insurance whatsoever, a judge can order rehab free to the average person seeking help.

Chapter 6

The Best Diet for Alcohol Detox

Eating may be the very last thing you'll need to take into consideration when it comes to alcohol consumption detoxification. But since alcohol consumption have an initial link together with your body's capacity to procedure and metabolize precise nourishment, you must begin to feed your body with the meals it requires to heal properly.

Through the original phases of the cleansing, it could be difficult to take any food whatsoever, but as your symptoms improve, it's necessary to consume a well-balanced diet that will aid in bringing your body back again to functional harmony.

Below covers what forms of foods, vitamins, and minerals you'll want associated with your daily diet during and after an alcohol cleansing.

Focus on Hydration

Through the original degrees of your alcohol cleanse,

remaining hydrated is incredibly essential. The beginning phases of the alcohol consumption drawback will generally induce some of the following symptoms:

- Fatigue
- Anxiety
- Nausea/vomiting
- Lack of appetite
- Depression

…and more.

Several symptoms will be worsened if you're also dehydrated. Since alcohol consumption dehydrate the body, you'll need to work doubly hard to be sure you give yourself a trusted supply of normal water. While you aren't thirsty, try to drink drinking water to greatly help flush your body of toxins.

Eat Soups And Fluids through the Preliminary Detox

When you beginning your alcohol detoxification, which frequently lasts which range from 24 and 72 hours, maybe it's challenging to keep food down. Don't pressure you to consume dense meals, actually if they are healthy ultimately. Instead, focus on consuming soups and other fluids to provide the body some extent of sustenance.

If you're preparing the soups yourself, make certain they include a large amount of vegetables, as well as low-fat resources of proteins, such as coffees, poultry, or seafood. You can even drink teas and fruits and veggie juices to maintain supply the body nutritional support.

Consist of Vitamin and Nutrient Support

Lots of people who are alcoholics commonly involve some vitamin and nutrient deficiencies. Alcohol consumption inhibit your body from effectively absorbing nutrition, including B supplements. B supplements are essential for changing food into functional energy. Common cleansing foods which contain B dietary vitamins include eggs, crazy, leafy greens, dairy, coffees, and fortified wholegrains.

Additional fat-soluble vitamins that you might be lacking include:

- Vitamin A (within fish, carrots, dairy)
- Vitamin D (inside the fortified dairy and fatty seafood)
- Vitamin E(within almonds, crazy, and natural vegetable oils)
- Vitamin K (within coconut oil, and leafy greens)

It's crucial to put an liquor nutrient program during your detox to have the ability to help your body heal and recover quicker.

Implement a Sensible Diet

Since alcohol consumption are heavy on sugars, it's common for folks detoxing from alcoholic drinks to crave sugary snacks and sweets. Try to reduce your using low-quality foods in support of well-balanced meals that support you on your own street to recovery. While you had been a comparatively healthy eater when you were consuming, alcoholic beverages nonetheless impair your body's capacity to utilize and breakdown essential nutrients.

A well-balanced diet carries a large amount of healthy vegetables & fruits, lean sources of proteins like fish and poultry, whole grains, nut products, coffees, and low-fat milk products. It's also vital that you add healthy oils such as coconut oil and essential coconut oil.

If you're choosing a remedy program to assist within your alcohol detox and recovery, you need to select a plan which includes dietary assistance and behavioral change within this program. This increase your recovery and ease your changeover to a recently sober life.

Types of Food to take when Detoxing from Alcohol

Withdrawal from alcohol consumption is different for everyone and may last from a few days to a complete week. However, the cleansing stage (every time a person is ridding oneself completely of alcohol consumption) can last good following the closing from the withdrawals, transporting on for two weeks. Much like the majority of situations in life, your body will react accordingly based on everything you placed involved with it with this stage.

When detoxing, you'll find out that first & most crucial is normal water. Hydration is essential generally, and particularly if withdrawing from alcohol consumption as the body is usually modifying to less liquid intake than typical. But certain food organizations likewise have benefits when it comes to the pain of withdrawals and detoxing. Another foods needed in the detoxification process.

1.   Fruits & vegetables

Because of the high degrees of fiber, fruits & vegetables will digest quickly. Additionally, people withdrawing or detoxing from alcohol consumption may often crave sweets. Fruits contain glucose, that may match the craving for something nice without weighing too greatly around the person's belly since appetite will decrease through the cleansing stage. Associated with Mayoclinic.com, some vegetables & fruits include raspberries, pears, oranges, strawberries, bananas, and figs.

2.   Whole grains

Carbohydrates are crucial for recovery, because they

offer soluble fiber and vigour that your detoxer could be lacking. Prepared grains such as white bread provide carbohydrates for energy but certainly are a less healthy option in the long-run. Wholegrain contains more fiber, leading to sense fuller instead of causing the body any digestive issues.

3.   Anything containing vitamin B

Continuous alcohol consumption leads to inadequate vitamin B. vitamin B is essential in the torso to replenish the body's supply. Foods high in vitamin B include salmon, broccoli, asparagus, and romaine lettuce.

4.   Proteins reduced fat

Many alcoholics in detoxification could have a lower life expectancy appetite or simply be powered down by food, but foods high in fiber might help them feel full. Protein with low fat content material is usually ideal because they favorably affect feeling and energy, leading to less prospect of relapse. Such foods include seafood and lean meat.

5.   Cayenne pepper

Though it could not sound appealing, adding cayenne pepper to foods can reduce alcohol cravings and increase appetite. That's helpful because in detoxification, the desire is commonly suppressed, and essential nutrients aren't received. Cayenne pepper may also help out with decreasing alcohol drawback symptoms such as nausea.

Though ensuring to consume these food types during detox won't ensure hanging out, they'll likely ease the discomfort and urges that accompany the detox stage.

Foods to avoid during Detox

- **Sugars**

Extreme sugar consumption causes prolonged cravings, lethargy, anxiety, and substance imbalances. Also, it often creates a fresh sort of addiction for folks in recovery.

- **Caffeine**

It overstimulates the central nervous system, that may bring about stress and insomnia, both which could be detrimental to effective cleansing and recovery.

Prepared or Processed foods

Because of this, the liver must work much harder to breakdown preservatives and chemicals within most of these foods, and in addition, you intend to let the liver to rest once you can during detoxification and early recovery.

Chapter 7

Natural Healthy Methods after Boozing'

Stay on the Wagon; Destination: Balance

America and arguably a big section of the world - is soaked in booze, making an alcohol cleansing challenging for those who dread they've crossed the collection between party and problem.

Predicated on the Countrywide Council on Alcoholism and Medicine Dependence (NCADD), alcohol consumption will be the most used addictive material in the U.S.: 17.6 million people, or one Atlanta divorce attorney (12 adults), is usually suffering from alcohol consumption mistreatment or dependence. For the time being, several million be a part of dangerous, binge consuming patterns. Virtually any interpersonal gathering revolves around booze, from frat celebrations to one-night time stands, making alcohol consumption difficult to withstand even though you realize that it's loaded with sugar and you will be offering no real benefits. Reducing or kicking your alcohol consumption habit ultimately could be necessary in repairing balance to your overall health and adding years to your lifestyle. Alcohol detox can help you do this.

Dangers of Alcohol Consumption

Alcohol consumption can directly harm the liver organ, intestines, digestive system, stomach, and oesophagus while increasing the likelihood of developing a laundry group of cancers, partly due to its high sugar content. Dr. Robert Lustig proved inside a 2015 report that sugar is "toxic no matter its calories and irrespective of its weight." When you consume alcohol, your body reacts to it like a toxin and throws its energy into eliminating it. Which means that additional processes are disrupted, including glucose production, especially in the liver as well as the hormones to modify it. Interfering using the liver's production of glucose could cause problems such as hypoglycemia. Alcohol also contains ethanol, a substance that may transform the mitochondrial structure, which plays an essential role in alcohol metabolism. Additionally, it could affect the function of several organs, just like the liver as well as the heart.

You don't need to drink a whole lot of alcohol because of this to have unwanted side effects. Actually moderate alcohol consumption can enhance the chance of breast cancer, promote mental decline, and impact pregnancy. For instance, pre-menopausal women who consume 10 ounces (just a little glass) of wine, an 8-ounce beer, or an ounce of hard liquor every day possess a 5 percent greater prospect of obtaining breast cancer. That number jumps to 9 percent for post-menopausal women, according to a written report from your American Institute for Cancer Research as well as the World Cancer Research Fund. So when you take these into consideration, roughly 12 percent of women in America and the United Kingdom could have breast cancer eventually within their lifetimes, that's a considerable increase in risk.

Furthermore, experts through the University of Oxford and London found that there's a relationship between moderate drinking and mental decline. Results of their 30-year study showed that folks who consumed high examples of alcohol were at an increased risk for Hippocampal atrophy, some sort of brain damage often connected with memory-loss circumstances like Alzheimer's and Dementia, which moderates that drinkers are 3times much more likely to own Hippocampal atrophy than individuals who didn't drink.

Another fresh research showed that consuming small amounts of alcohol when pregnant could change a child's features. Experts discovered that alcohol consumption affected face shape, specifically round the nose, eyes, and lips, when consumed through the entire pregnancy and in the first trimester.

Why Alcohol Detox?

Despite its dangers, moderate and heavy alcohol consumption is sticking around. In 2015, Millennial drank a lot more than 42 percent of all wine in the U.S., according to a written report from your own wine Market Council. Even the rise in popularity and legalization of recreational marijuana in the U.S. hasn't negatively impacted alcohol consumption and sales. Colorado tax records show that both developed a pseudo symbiotic relationship, steadily increasing side-by-side.

If the "one drink" often becomes 3 or 4, you may be

damaging your pancreas, tampering together with your body's sugar levels, reducing communication between your brain plus your body, developing an emotional or physical dependency, putting yourself vulnerable to developing liver disease, and more. You may be putting some nasty toxins within you. For example, a report found that 14 popular German beers are filled up with glyphosate, the active component in Monsanto's weed-killer Roundup, and it's likely within other beers that have not been investigated.

Natural Alcohol Cleansing Methods

So, what can we do to fight the results of constant alcohol consumption? Everything starts with alcohol detox. That is done in a hospital, but you're guaranteed to be pumped with medications that are cross-tolerant with alcohol you need to include their band of risks such as benzodiazepines (anti-anxiety medications) and anticonvulsants. Thankfully, nature has come through for all those once again giving incredible herbs, plants, vitamins, and minerals like passionflower, milk thistle, vitamin B, and activated charcoal that facilitate an all-natural alcohol detox process. Another strategies don't reverse the damage of ongoing alcoholism; however, they are able to kick beginning your overall health journey, whether you intend to:

·   Overcome a hangover

·   Scale backwards on occasional drinking

·   End binge drinking

·   End consuming completely

For individuals who drink occasionally or want to remove a hangover, concentrate on numbers two, three, five, and ten below. For all people targeting alcohol withdrawal symptoms from binge drinking, concentrate on numbers one, eight, and six. If you're trying to stop completely, pay special concentrate on numbers four, five, seven, and nine. Never try to detox without medical supervision. An expert will help you decide on what's best for your body, and which combination of alcohol detox methods are best for you personally.

Listed below are ten (10) natural alcohol detoxification methods:

1. Drink Passion Blossom Tea

Many people experience insomnia and anxiety during an alcohol detox because when the body undergoes a withdrawal of alcohol, a substance used to operate with, which is often utilized to self-medicate anxiety, the mind starts young chemicals and neurotransmitters that put extra stress on your own brain function. Ultimately, this leads to anxiety, that may cause restlessness and disrupted sleep patterns.

Drinking flower tea or passionflower extract can enhance the quality of slumber and anxiety levels. Research means that passionflower is definitely an efficient treatment for insomnia, so when in conjunction with herbs like valerian, hops, and lemon balm is a lot more efficient. Top-quality products such as they are from Native Remedies Pure Calm (with passionflower, lemon balm and lavender (with passionflower, kava, and St. John's Wort) aswell for sound sleep:

Another study found that enthusiasm blossom helped

alleviate anxiety connected with alcohol consumption withdrawals. When analysts offered alcohol-addicted mice experiencing withdrawals interest flower extract, the mice's withdrawal anxiety was reduced by 90 percent compared to mice that didn't experience the extract.

2. Essential Oils

The first stages of the cleansing process will most likely include fighting withdrawal. Janice Rosenthal, who owns your garden of Essences and aromatherapy expert, suggests organic essential oils to soothe your experience. She recommends mixing 15 drops of body butter and putting it to your upper abdomen, sides, and rear. That is clearly a powerful do-it-yourself solution, which works rapidly to detoxify the liver, as the essential oils permeate your skin layer and reach the liver's bloodstream directly within around thirty minutes," Rosenthal explains.

3. B-complex vitamins

Alcohol consumption could cause your body to melt away through B vitamins quicker than normal. Replenishing your body with B-complex supplements like B-1, B-3, and B-5 reduces alcohol withdrawal symptoms and supports the detoxification process. Research demonstrates vitamin B-1, a vitamin that alcoholics are usually deficient in.

It could lessen fatigue and increase effective brain functioning, while vitamin B-5 helps eliminate alcohol within you and supports adrenal function. According to Dr. Alex Roher, M.D., vitamin B-3 may also relieve the symptoms of alcohol withdrawal like cravings and insomnia. "Niacin (vitamin B-3) could be especially effective in larger recommended doses," Roher says.

4. Activated Charcoal

Fired up charcoal is a robust vitamin that works to capture chemicals and toxins in the body, rendering it an excellent detoxifier. Qualified Nutritional Specialist, Renee Belz, highly recommends activated charcoal for detoxing from alcohol. "My absolute No.1 (alcohol detox vitamin) is charcoal. It binds toxins in the GI tract (especially alcohol)," she says.

Belz claims that activated charcoal works well before and after consuming alcohol. However, studies show that it could considerably reduce blood alcohol concentrations when taken at the same time as alcohol. Belz says that typical protocol demands 1,000 to 2,000 mg of activated charcoal.

5. Bring Milk Thistle

Milk thistle established the actual fact to be an all-natural liver organ detoxifier and it is often recommended as an all-natural fix for alcohol consumption detoxification. Although, research means that milk thistle may regenerate damaged liver tissue, remove poisons in the body, and block the absorption of alcohol in the liver. Belz explains that milk thistle dosage varies based on bodyweight, however the typical protocol is 50 mg from the powerful liver detoxifier. You are able to consume the milk thistle plant's leaves and seeds in powder, pill, tea, tincture, or extract form. Liver tonics with milk thistle being a primary ingredient, provide comprehensive liver detoxification.

6. Devote a Dash of Cayenne

Adding cayenne pepper to your meal or taking a single drop dose can help alleviate alcohol withdrawal symptoms. Dr. Samuel Malloy, director at DrFelix and expert in holistic medicine, recommends cayenne pepper for common symptoms. "Cayenne pepper may increase your appetite, and it includes unpleasant withdrawal symptoms like nausea," says Malloy.

"Additionally, it could reduce the pain of any tummy problems because of drinking excessive degrees of alcohol, because it's high in anti-inflammatory substances." Cayenne pepper may also reduce inflammation from the stomach lining that's due to excessive alcohol consumption. Take a look in its natural, powdered, cream, or capsule form to reap advantages of its detoxifying properties!

7. Advantages from Kudzu

Kudzu main is a standard Chinese herb that's traditionally within Japan and Southeast Asia to lessen various side effects of excessive alcohol consumption (hangovers, thirst, etc.). However, recent research demonstrates kudzu root vitamins, that are filled with strong antioxidants referred to as phytochemicals, that may curb alcohol cravings. A placebo-controlled double-blind human study found that participants who received kudzu root drank a significantly fewer level of beers than those that received the placebo.

Its antioxidant properties may also lessen overall liver harm and regenerate damaged liver organ. One study demonstrated that kudzu root extract stimulated liver regeneration and made the liver more resistant in adult male rats put through a chemical that creates liver toxicity (carbon tetrachloride). In the event that you don't need to contemplate it like a vitamin, take a look being a powder. Sneak it in to the following sauce or soup!

8. Try Robuvit - French Oak Wooden Extract

Natural health physician and author Dr. Fred Pescatore, suggests a French oak wood extract, as an all-natural way to detox from alcohol. Research means that Robuvit helps support the liver's natural detox function through the elimination of poisons faster. Pescatore says that "if we consume alcohol, the short-term overload may exceed the liver's capacity to process and filter, that may result in the normal "hangover" effects the majority are familiar with." A fresh research demonstrates Robuvit® really helps to protect the liver from alcohol-related damage and "to significantly improve symptoms of short-term hepatic damage including fatigue, nausea, and mild liver enlargement," Pescatore says. "It's safe, easy, and effective."

9. Angelica Extract

Angelica extract is a robust anti-inflammatory plant that will help reduce alcohol cravings and relieve withdrawal symptoms like headaches and bloating. It's also an antispasmodic agent, which smooth muscle spasms (particularly in the gastrointestinal tract), assisting the liver and spleen during long-term alcohol users' recovery processes. three to five 5 drops in a single glass of water usually does the trick. Be cautious with this one. Angelica extract can make you sick or nauseous in the event that you get back to drinking.

10. Agua

It's quite crucial to stay hydrated during any detox. Water really helps to flush out the poisons in the body, replenish your body's drinking water amounts, and lessen the intensity of symptoms like withdrawal-related headaches. Try mixing in a few lemon juices to improve your alcohol detox. Lemon water offers a wholesome supply of vitamin C, helps restore your pH balance, and even more. You may try coconut drinking water. It adds alkalinity to your body, and it's full of potassium and various other electrolytes and nutrients that may soothe an upset stomach or nausea.

CPSIA information can be obtained
at www.ICGtesting.com
Printed in the USA
LVHW051257231220
674977LV00001B/125